MATERNITY & WOMEN'S HEALTH NCLEX-RN REVIEW:

100 Practice Questions with Detailed Rationales Explaining Correct & Incorrect Answer Choices

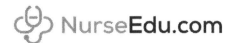

Disclaimer:

Although the author and publisher have made every effort to ensure that the information in this book was correct at press time, the author and publisher do not assume and hereby disclaim any liability to any party for any loss, damage, or disruption caused by errors or omissions, whether such errors or omissions result from negligence, accident, or any other cause.

This book is not intended as a substitute for the medical advice of physicians. The reader should regularly consult a physician in matters relating to their health and particularly with respect to any symptoms that may require diagnosis or medical attention.

NCLEX®, NCLEX®-RN, and NCLEX®-PN are registered trademarks of the National Council of State Boards of Nursing, Inc. They hold no affiliation with this product.

Some images within this book are either royalty-free images, used under license from their respective copyright holders, or images that are in the public domain.

ISBN: 978-1-952914-14-0

FREE BONUS

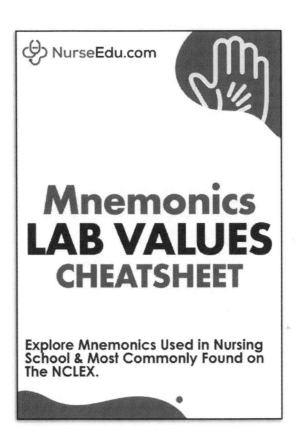

FREE Download – Just Visit:

NurseEdu.com/bonus

TABLE OF CONTENTS

CHAPTER 1:

NCLEX-RN – MATERNITY: PRENATAL - 25 QUESTIONS

1. The nurse is preparing a teaching session for women who are planning to become pregnant. Which preconception health measures should be taken within the 3 months prior to conception should be included in this teaching plan? Select all that apply.

   A. Smoking cessation
   B. Take daily vitamins that include 4 mg of folic acid
   C. Get the rubella vaccine if blood testing shows the presence of rubella IgG antibodies
   D. Develop an exercise regime
   E. Get the annual influenza vaccine

   Rationale:

   Correct answer: A, B, D, E

As smoking represents serious risks for the mother and fetus, such as placenta previa, preterm rupture of membranes, and pregnancy loss, women who are planning to become pregnant should take steps to stop smoking if possible, or limit cigarette use as much as possible. The Institute of Medicine recommends that women of childbearing age take 4 mg of folic acid per day before conception, then 6 mg per day while pregnant. Women are advised to develop a regular exercise plan at least 3 months prior to becoming pregnant to provide aerobic conditioning and general muscle toning. A new exercise regime should not be started after conception. Women who plan to become pregnant should receive their annual flu vaccine.

C is incorrect. The presence of rubella IgG antibodies indicates the woman is immune to rubella, either due to previous infection with rubella or previous vaccination. *Absence* of rubella IgG antibodies indicates lack of immunity. Women who are not immune to rubella should be counseled regarding the risks of infection during the first trimester. They should delay conception for three months if they do receive the vaccine, as the vaccine is a live attenuated virus preparation and can be teratogenic to the fetus.

2. The nurse is planning topics to be addressed during prenatal education classes for women in the first trimester of pregnancy. Which topics should be discussed during this period? Select all that apply.

    A. Preparation for the birth process
    B. Benefits of breastfeeding
    C. Choosing a pediatrician
    D. Relaxation techniques
    E. Foods to avoid during pregnancy

Rationale:

Correct answer: B, C, E.

Topics to be addressed in the first trimester of pregnancy include, in part, issues such as infant feeding options and the benefits of breastfeeding, guidelines for choosing a pediatrician to provide care for the newborn, and foods to avoid during pregnancy (sushi and other raw fish, undercooked meat, poultry and eggs, and unpasteurized products).

A and D are incorrect. Information regarding preparation for the birth process and relaxation and breathing techniques are addressed beginning in the second trimester of pregnancy.

3. The nurse informs a female patient that the results of a blood test indicate the presence of human chorionic gonadotropin [hCG]. The nurse recognizes this positive pregnancy test result represents which type of changes that are signs of pregnancy?

    A. Presumptive changes
    B. Objective changes
    C. Subjective changes
    D. Diagnostic changes

Rationale:

Correct answer: B

A positive result for a clinical pregnancy lab test is considered an objective, or probable, sign of pregnancy. Objective or probable signs include physiologic changes in the woman's body that can be observed by the examiner, including elevation in basal body temperature, clinical lab tests, over-the-counter pregnancy tests, and observable changes in internal pelvic organs. The presence of these objective changes does not represent a definitive diagnosis of pregnancy.

A, C, and D are incorrect. Presumptive signs of pregnancy consist of symptoms the woman experiences, such as morning sickness, breast changes, fatigue, amenorrhea or urinary frequency. Subjective changes are based on individual opinions and perceptions and are not valid in determining the presence of a pregnancy. Diagnostic changes that are definitively positive signs of pregnancy are the fetal heartbeat (audible with a doppler at 10 weeks of gestation), fetal movement palpated by the examiner, and visualization of the fetus by ultrasound or x-ray.

4. The nurse is providing care for a woman in the prenatal clinic who is unsure about the date of her last menstrual period [LMP], as her periods were irregular. The nurse recognizes that the following factors will help to determine the estimated date of birth [EDB], and indicate the potential viability of the pregnancy, with which exception?

    A. Evaluation of uterine size
    B. Ultrasound exam within the first 30 days of gestation
    C. Auscultation of the fetal heartrate
    D. Establishing when quickening occurs or did occur

Rationale:

Correct answer: B

Research data indicate that while routine diagnostic ultrasound can be used to help determine the EDB, scans that are done before 40 days of gestation are not useful.

A is incorrect because evaluation of uterine size can help determine the EDB when the LMP is in question.

C is incorrect because auscultation of the fetal heart rate is a reliable method of determining EDB. First semester normal fetal heart rate is generally between 110-170 beats per minute.

D is incorrect because determining the date of quickening can also help identify the EDB when the LMP is in question. Quickening can start as early as 13 weeks but is not expected until 20-25 weeks. A, C, and D are positive changes associated with the normal progression of pregnancy.

5. The patient in the prenatal clinic indicates that the first day of her last menstrual period [LMP] was November 8th. Using Naegele's rule, the estimated date of birth [EDB] will be on which month and day of the following year.

   A. August 8
   B. August 15
   C. August 11
   D. July 15

Rationale:

Correct answer: B

Using Naegele's rule, the EDB for this patient will be on August 15 of the following year. Naegele's rule = First day of LMP [November 8] - 3 months [August 8] + 7 days = EDB of August 15. The resulting EDB is approximately 280 days from the LMP.

A, C, and D are incorrect calculations.

6. A patient in the prenatal clinic was screened for gestational diabetes mellitus at 28 weeks' gestation. After an hour, the result of this screening was a blood glucose of 120 mg/dL. What follow-up is indicated?

    A. An immediate 100-gram 3 hour glucose tolerance test [OGTT]
    B. Assessment of long-term glucose control
    C. A 100-gram 3-hour OGTT in 3 - 4 days
    D. No further assessment is needed

Rationale:

Correct answer: D

A blood glucose level under 130 mg/dL is a normal response to the screening test of a 1 hour, 50-gram oral glucose challenge test and does not indicate the need for further follow-up for this issue.

A is incorrect because, if needed, OGTT testing would be done at least 3 days later, as the patient must consume at least 150 grams of carbohydrate per day for at least 3 days before the test is done.

B is incorrect because the screening results are normal, requiring no further follow up.

C is incorrect because the OGTT test is only needed if the gestational diabetes screening shows glucose greater than 130 mg/dL.

7. When assessing a patient at 18 weeks' gestation, the nurse notes a decrease in blood pressure from the previous baseline levels. Which nursing action is indicated?

    A. Document as a normal finding
    B. Notify the certified nurse-midwife
    C. Assess for signs of orthostatic hypotension
    D. Retake the blood pressure

Rationale:

Correct answer: A

The nurse should expect to observe a decrease in the patient's blood pressure from the previous baseline during the second trimester related to normal physiologic changes. Documentation is the appropriate nursing action when findings are normal.

B is incorrect because the healthcare provider does not need to be notified of expected findings.

C is incorrect because assessment for orthostatic hypotension is only indicated if the patient experiences specific symptoms, such as dizziness or transient black spots in front of the eyes when changing positions, for instance, from sitting to standing up.

D is incorrect because reassessment of the blood pressure is not needed as this is an expected finding.

8. During the first prenatal visit, the nurse reviews danger signs in pregnancy with the patient. These signs include... Select all that apply.

   A. Suprapubic pressure prior to 37 weeks' gestation
   B. Frequent urination during the first 12 weeks of pregnancy
   C. Epigastric discomfort during the 2nd and 3rd trimesters
   D. Recurring, transient low back pain beginning at 34 weeks' gestation

Rationale:

Correct answer: A, D

Danger signs associated with preterm labor include, in part, suprapubic pain or pressure and low, dull back pain.

B is incorrect. Urinary frequency is a common discomfort occurring in the first three and last three months of pregnancy. As the uterus grows, it places pressure on the bladder.

C is incorrect. Pregnant women may experience epigastric pain, or heartburn, due to relaxation of stomach muscles and food backing up into the lower esophagus. The stomach may also produce more acid during pregnancy. In addition, the growing baby pressing against the stomach can force acid upward causing heartburn.

9. The nurse is caring for a patient in the prenatal clinic who is experiencing nausea and vomiting of pregnancy [NVP]. Self-care measures such as small, frequent meals and drinking carbonated beverages have been only moderately effective. Which additional measures can be suggested?

    A. Take 250 mg ginger capsules four times per day
    B. Take doxylamine 12.5 mg each morning
    C. Drink black tea with sugar three times per day
    D. Take vitamin B6 25 mg daily with prenatal vitamins

Rationale:

Correct answer: A

Over-the-counter preparations that have been found to be effective for mild-to-moderate NVP include 250 mg ginger tablets taken four times a day (pregnant women should not exceed 1 g of ginger per day).

B is incorrect because doxylamine causes drowsiness and should be taken at bedtime.

C is incorrect because black tea contains caffeine, which should be limited during pregnancy, and sugary beverages can worsen nausea.

D is incorrect because the typical dose of vitamin B6 for nausea during pregnancy is 25 mg three times a day, rather than once a day. The pregnant woman should not exceed 100 mg of vitamin B6 daily, as this can cause nerve damage.

10. Following a discussion related to alcohol use during pregnancy, which statement by the patient indicates the patient has the correct understanding about the information provided?

    A. "Since I am past the first trimester, I can occasionally have some wine with dinner."
    B. "It is safe to drink moderately in the last few weeks of pregnancy."
    C. "I will abstain from using alcohol while I am pregnant."

D. "Beverages such as ale or beer are safe in small amounts."

Rationale:

Correct answer: C

The CDC and the U.S. Surgeon General state, "There is no known safe amount of alcohol to drink while pregnant. There is also no safe time during pregnancy to drink and no safe kind of alcohol." Similarly, the American Academy of Pediatrics advises, "There is no safe amount of alcohol when a woman is pregnant. Evidence based research states that even drinking small amounts of alcohol while pregnant can lead to miscarriage, stillbirth, prematurity, or sudden infant death syndrome."

A, B, and D are incorrect as they indicate the idea that there is a safe level of use of alcohol during pregnancy.

11. The nurse is caring for a woman in the prenatal clinic who has a body mass index [BMI] of 26 and is concerned about weight gain associated with this pregnancy. What are the recommendations for weight gain during pregnancy for this patient?

   A. Total weight gain 28 - 40 pounds, gaining 1 - 1.3 pounds per week after the first trimester

B. Total weight gain 15 - 25 pounds, gaining 0.5 - 0.7 pounds per week after the first trimester

C. Total weight gain 25 - 35 pounds, gaining 0.8 - 1 pounds per week after the first trimester

D. Total weight gain 11 - 20 pounds, gaining 0.4 - 0.6 pounds per week after the first trimester

Rationale:

Correct answer: B

BMI is body mass in kg divided by height in meters squared. The woman's BMI of 26 indicates she is overweight. (Normal BMI is 18.5-25 kg/m^2). Recommendations for weight gain during pregnancy for overweight women are a total weight gain of 15 - 25 pounds, gaining 0.5 - 0.7 pounds per week in the second and third trimester.

A is incorrect because this is the recommendation for women who are underweight.

C is incorrect because this is the recommendation for women who are at a normal weight.

D is incorrect because this the recommendation for women who are obese.

12. A woman who has just learned that she is pregnant is concerned about her recent decision to adopt a vegetarian

diet. Which statement regarding a vegetarian diet during pregnancy is correct?

A. A vegan diet cannot adequately provide nutrients needed during pregnancy.
B. Well-planned vegetarian diets can be nutritionally adequate during pregnancy.
C. A vegetarian diet will increase the risk for a low-birth-weight infant.
D. A strict vegan diet will provide all the nutrients needed to support pregnancy.

Rationale:

Correct answer: B.

Well-planned vegetarian diets are nutritionally adequate and appropriate during all stages of life, including pregnancy. The key is in "well-planned," recognizing that some added vitamins or supplements may be needed. For example, if the diet includes fewer than four servings of milk and dairy foods, calcium supplementation may be necessary.

A is incorrect because a vegan diet can provide the necessary nutrients if B12 is taken daily.

C is incorrect because, as stated, with appropriate meal planning, a vegetarian diet is not necessarily a risk factor for low birth weight. It must be recognized that meal-planning *must* include needed vitamins and supplements and provide adequate caloric intake.

D is incorrect because a vegan diet lacks animal products, and thus, the pregnant woman on this diet is at risk of vitamin B12 deficiency. The nurse must teach the pregnant vegan patient about the need for B12 fortified foods (available products include fortified soy and rice beverages and some breakfast cereals), or she may require a daily supplement of vitamin B12. A vegan diet can *only* provide the nutritional needs if B12 is specifically accounted for in daily food choices or supplementation.

13. The nurse is caring for a patient in the prenatal clinic who has asked about using artificial sweeteners. Which statement regarding the use of artificial sweeteners is correct?

    A. Sweeteners such as aspartame must be avoided during pregnancy.

    B. Only natural sweeteners, such as stevia sweeteners, should be used during pregnancy.

    C. Cyclamate is safe to use during pregnancy.

    D. Sweeteners considered safe during pregnancy include aspartame and sucralose.

Rationale:

Correct answer: D.

Sweeteners that are classified by the Food and Drug Administration as Generally Recognized as Safe [GRAS], are acceptable for use during pregnancy. These include aspartame (Equal or NutraSweet), sucralose (Splenda), and acesulfame potassium (Sunett).

A is incorrect because aspartame is safe to use during pregnancy. It is often found as an additive to soft drinks, gelatin, desserts, pudding mixes, beverages, chewing gum, and dairy products.

B is incorrect because some non-natural sweeteners are safe to use during pregnancy, as well as stevia.

C is incorrect because cyclamate, formerly used as an artificial sweetener, is banned for use in the US.

14. The nurse identifies that the serum glucose levels for a pregnant woman who has completed a 100-gram 3-hour oral glucose tolerance [OGTT] test are: Fasting: 90 mg/dL, 1 hour: 185 mg/dL, 2 hours: 155 mg/dL, 3 hours: 135 mg/dL. What is the significance of these findings?

    A. The serum glucose levels are within normal limits for a woman during pregnancy.
    B. The test results indicate a medical diagnosis of gestational diabetes.

C. Gestational diabetes can be ruled out, as the 3 hour serum glucose levels are below 140 mg/dL.

D. The test results indicate that the patient should be further screened by testing glycosylated hemoglobin [HbA1c] levels.

Rationale:

Correct answer: B

Gestational diabetes is diagnosed if two or more of the following serum glucose levels for OGTT screening are met or exceeded: Fasting: 95 mg/dL, 1 hour: 180 mg/dL, 2 hours: 155 mg/dL, 3 hours: 140 mg/dL. The patient's results meet or exceed two of the four listed.

A is incorrect because the patient's results include elevated serum glucose levels at 1 and 2 hours, which are not within normal limits for pregnancy.

C is incorrect because even though the fasting and 3-hour levels are within normal limits, the presence of two abnormal levels indicate gestational diabetes.

D is incorrect because HbA1c level testing is not reliable for screening for gestational diabetes. HbA1c is used to determine average blood glucose control in non-pregnant patients over the last 2-3 months.

15. A pregnant woman has come to the emergency department reporting vaginal bleeding, cramping, and back ache. A pelvic exam reveals that the cervix has dilated. These signs are consistent with which type of spontaneous abortion?

    A. Threatened abortion
    B. Imminent abortion
    C. Incomplete abortion
    D. Missed abortion

Rationale:

Correct answer: B

An imminent (inevitable) abortion is characterized by bleeding and cramping and dilation of the cervical os. Typically, the placenta has begun to detach from the uterine wall, and membranes may rupture.

A is incorrect. A threatened abortion is characterized by vaginal bleeding within the first 20 weeks of pregnancy. The cervical os is typically closed rather than dilated, and miscarriage is a possibility.

C is incorrect. An incomplete abortion involves dilation of the cervical os and expulsion of the embryo/fetus with some retained products of conception, often the placenta, remaining in the uterus.

D is incorrect. With a missed abortion, the cervix is closed. Uterine growth stops, breast changes regress, and the woman may have a brownish vaginal discharge. If the fetus is retained inside the uterus longer than 6 weeks, disseminated intravascular coagulation may develop.

16. A patient calls the prenatal clinic with concerns about vaginal bleeding. Which additional information would indicate a potential for spontaneous abortion? Select all that apply.

    A. Pelvic cramping
    B. Fever
    C. Backache
    D. Braxton-Hicks contractions
    E. Fetal heartrate 120-160 bpm

Rationale:

Correct answer: A, C

The more reliable indicators of a potential spontaneous abortion are the presence of pelvic cramping and backache. These symptoms are usually absent with bleeding related to polyps, ruptured cervical blood vessels, or cervical erosion.

B is incorrect because while febrile illness may increase the risk for spontaneous abortion, fever is not a symptom associated with spontaneous abortion itself.

D is incorrect because Braxton-Hicks contractions are sporadic uterine contractions, thought to be an aid in preparing the body for birth. They are not dangerous and are not related to spontaneous abortion.

E is incorrect because this is within the normal range for fetal heartrate and is not an indication of spontaneous abortion.

17. The nurse is assessing a patient who is at 27 weeks' gestation in the prenatal clinic. She was of normal weight before pregnancy, with no significant prior medical history. Which assessment findings should be reported to the physician immediately? Select all that apply.

    A. Dizziness
    B. Swollen ankles
    C. Moderate facial edema
    D. Weight gain 1 pound from the previous week
    E. Blurred vision

Rationale:

Correct answer: C, E.

Moderate facial edema and blurred vision is consistent with preeclampsia, which must be reported to the healthcare provider. Other symptoms characteristic of preeclampsia include headache, oliguria, RUQ pain, and proteinuria greater than 300 mg/dL per 24 h.

A is incorrect because dizziness during pregnancy is a common symptom, which may be caused by low blood pressure due to the uterus compressing major arteries, low blood sugar, low iron, quickly moving from a sitting position to a standing position, or dehydration.

B is incorrect because this is an expected finding. Edema in the lower extremities is a common occurrence during pregnancy, associated with decreased venous return from the legs due to pressure on pelvic veins and the vena cava by the growing uterus.

D is incorrect because this is a normal finding. Women of normal pre-pregnancy weight are expected to gain a total of 25 - 35 pounds over the course of the pregnancy, gaining 0.8 - 1 pound per week after the first trimester. Weight gain of 2 pounds in a week during the second trimester may be an indication of pregnancy induced hypertension, or pre-eclampsia.

18. When assessing a patient in the prenatal clinic, which assessment findings indicate the presence of possible complications? Select all that apply.

   A. Epigastric pain
   B. Blurred vision
   C. Dependent edema
   D. Proteinuria
   E. Nausea
   F. Dark skin blotches on cheeks

Rationale:

Correct answer: A, B, D

Signs of severe preeclampsia include, in part, visual disturbances such as blurred vision, epigastric, or right upper quadrant abdominal pain, and protein in the urine. These signs indicate end-organ effects of preeclampsia.

C is incorrect because edema in the lower extremities is a common occurrence during pregnancy associated with decreased venous return from the legs due to pressure on pelvic veins and the vena cava by the growing uterus. However, a sudden increase in swelling, especially in the face and hands, may be associated with preeclampsia.

E is incorrect because nausea is common due to hormonal changes, especially during the first trimester of pregnancy.

F is incorrect because darkened skin blotches on the forehead and cheeks, known as the "mask of pregnancy" is common due to increased pigmentation during pregnancy. A similar-colored darkened vertical line on the abdomen may be seen as well (linea nigra).

19. The nurse is caring for a patient in the prenatal clinic at 12 weeks' gestation who is experiencing vaginal bleeding. Arrange the following descriptions of the categories related to the progression of types of spontaneous abortion. All options must be used.

   A. Bleeding and cramping increase; the internal cervical os dilates; membranes may rupture.
   B. All products of conception are expelled. The cervical os may be closed.
   C. Bleeding, cramping, and backache; the cervical os is closed.
   D. Uterine growth ceases; breast changes regress. The cervix is closed.
   E. Part of the products of conception are retained; the cervical os is dilated.

   Rationale:

   Correct answer order: C, A, E, B, D

C describes a threatened abortion, characterized by unexplained bleeding, pelvic cramping, and backache. The cervix is closed. This condition may resolve without threat to the fetus or may progress to partial or complete expulsion of pregnancy.

A describes the next classification, an imminent (or inevitable) abortion, characterized by increased bleeding and cramping and dilation of the cervical os. Membranes may rupture at this stage.

E describes an incomplete abortion, where part of the products of conception is retained in the uterus, typically the placenta. The internal cervical os is dilated.

B describes a complete abortion, where all products of conception are expelled, the uterus is contracted, and the cervical os may be closed.

D describes a missed abortion. In this situation, fetal demise has occurred, but the fetus is not expelled. Uterine growth ceases, breast changes regress, and the cervix is closed. The woman may have a brownish vaginal discharge.

*Tip: on the NCLEX exam, these answers will be presented on the left side of the screen, and the student will have to drag them to the right side of the screen and place them in the correct order. No partial credit is given on the NCLEX, so all the answers must be in the exact correct order to get the question correct.

20. When assessing a patient in the prenatal clinic who is at 16 weeks' gestation, which of these findings would indicate a potential complication of pregnancy?

    A. Fundal height measurement of 20 cm.
    B. Sporadic uterine contractions
    C. Decrease in blood pressure from the previous baseline
    D. Transient pain that travels down one side into the groin area

Rationale:

Correct answer: A

Uterine enlargement greater than expected for gestational age is a classic sign of hydatidiform mole (gestational trophoblastic disease), caused by degeneration of chorionic villi. When a patient presents with this condition, hCG levels will be elevated, no fetal heart tones will be heard, and the patient may experience a small amount of dark red-brown vaginal bleeding with passage of small, grapelike clusters.

B is incorrect. This describes Braxton-Hicks contractions: common and expected sporadic "false" uterine contractions that are usually felt in the second trimester or third trimester of pregnancy.

C is incorrect because the nurse should expect to observe a decrease in the patient's blood pressure from the previous baseline during the second trimester related to normal physiologic changes.

D is incorrect because this describes round ligament pain. The round ligaments are two cord-like bands that connect to the top of the uterus and run down to the low pelvic sidewall. As the uterus grows during pregnancy, these ligaments stretch and thicken to accommodate and provide support. These changes may occasionally cause pain on one or both sides, typically first noticed during the second trimester.

21. The nurse has given a patient in the prenatal clinic instructions about how to perform a daily count of fetal movements. Which statement by the patient indicates a need for further instruction?

   A. "I will use a clock and record the number of times I feel the baby move."
   B. "It is best to lie on my back and place my hands on the largest part of my abdomen."
   C. "I should perform the fetal movement counts at the same time each day."

D. "It is best to count the baby's movements after a meal, or after a short walk."

Rationale:

Correct answer: B

The woman should lie on her side, rather than on her back. She should rest in a quiet place with no distractions, place her hands on the largest part of her abdomen, and concentrate on fetal movements.

A is incorrect because it indicates understanding of the instructions. Fewer than three fetal movements in a one-hour period should be reported to the healthcare provider.

C is incorrect because no need for further education is needed related to this patient statement.

D is incorrect because it represents an appropriate understanding of the way to perform fetal movement counts. Fetal movement is most likely to be felt after the mom has ingested a meal or been physically active.

22. The nurse is assessing a patient in the prenatal clinic who is at 32 weeks' gestation. Ultrasound examination shows that the fetus is in a left occiput-anterior (LOA) position. To assess the fetal heart rate, the nurse would expect to

hear fetal heart sounds in which area of the woman's abdomen?

A. On the right side of the mother's abdomen

B. At the mother's midline

C. At or above the level of the umbilicus

D. Left lower quadrant, away from the midline

Rationale:

Correct answer: D

With the fetal in left occiput-anterior position, the baby is vertex, with the occiput of the baby's head facing anteriorly on the mother's left side. Fetal heart sounds will be heard in the left lower abdominal quadrant, below the level of the umbilicus, away from the mother's midline.

A is incorrect because when the baby is in LOA presentation, fetal heart sounds will be heard on the left side of the mother's abdomen.

B is incorrect because when the baby is in LOA presentation, fetal heart sounds will be heard on the left side of the mother's abdomen.

C is incorrect because fetal heart sounds will be heard at or above the umbilicus level when the fetus is in a breech or a sacral-anterior position.

23. The maternal serum alpha-fetoprotein [MSAFP] level for a woman at 18 weeks' gestation is 32 MoM [multiple of the median]. The nurse is aware that this MSAFP level is associated with which possible defects/ anomalies? Select all that apply.

    A. Down syndrome
    B. Congenital nephrosis
    C. Anencephaly
    D. Gestational trophoblastic disease
    E. Abdominal wall defects

Rationale:

Correct answer: B, C, E

The normal range for MSFAP is 0.5 - 2.5 MoM. Elevated AFP levels are associated with birth defects such as open neural tube defects, open abdominal wall defects, and congenital nephrosis. Elevations are also associated with Rh isoimmunization, multiple gestation, maternal diabetes mellitus, and fetoplacental dysfunction.

A incorrect because decreased MSFAP levels are associated with Down syndrome.

D is incorrect because gestational trophoblastic disease (or trisomy 18) is indicated by decreased MSFAP, not increased.

24. A patient in the prenatal clinic at 26 weeks' gestation is scheduled to have an ultrasound examination. The nurse understands that this ultrasound is done for which purpose(s)? Select all that apply.

   A. Diagnose fetal sickle-cell anemia
   B. Identify fetal position and presentation
   C. Assess lecithin-sphingomyelin ratio
   D. Determine the Biophysical Profile score
   E. Evaluate quickening

Rationale:

Correct answer: B, D

This patient is in the second trimester of pregnancy. Ultrasound during the second and third trimesters are done, in part, to identify fetal position and presentation and to determine the Biophysical Profile score.

A is incorrect because fetal sickle-cell anemia is diagnosed by chorionic villi sampling, done between 8-12 weeks' gestation. Ultrasound does not diagnose fetal sickle-cell anemia.

C is incorrect because lecithin-sphingomyelin ratio is assessed by amniocentesis (around 30 weeks' gestation) to determine lung maturity. This cannot be assessed by ultrasound.

E is incorrect because quickening is reported by the patient, not evaluated by ultrasound.

25. A contraction stress test [CST] done at 32 weeks' gestation is classified as negative. Which of the following describes a negative CST result?

    A. Late decelerations of the fetal heart rate with > 50% of uterine contractions

    B. Late decelerations of the fetal heart rate with < 50% of uterine contractions

    C. Quality of tracing inadequate to assess or less than three contractions in 10 minutes

    D. Three uterine contractions in 10 minutes without late decelerations of the fetal heart rate

Rationale:

Correct answer: D

A negative CST is a normal and reassuring test result, indicated by three uterine contractions in 10 minutes, lasting 40-60 seconds, without late decelerations of the fetal heart rate.

A is incorrect because this describes a positive, non-reassuring, abnormal test result.

B is incorrect because this describes a suspicious or equivocal test result. The test should be repeated in 24 hours.

C is incorrect because this describes an unsatisfactory test result. The test should be repeated in 24 hours.

CHAPTER 2:

NCLEX-RN – MATERNITY: MATERNAL INFANT HEALTH - 50 QUESTIONS

1. The clinic nurse is taking the history of a female patient who has missed her period. The urinalysis comes back positive for pregnancy, and the patient reports that her last missed period was on July 16, 2016. Using Naegele's Rule, the nurse would chart the patient's estimated delivery date as:

   A. April 16, 2017
   B. May 26, 2017
   C. April 23, 2017
   D. April 30, 2017

Rationale:

Correct answer: C

According to Naegele's Rule, this patient's estimated date of delivery would be April 23, 2017. To use Naegele's Rule, the nurse should take the patient's first day of her last missed period and add nine months and seven days.

July 16 + nine months = April 16

April 16 + seven days = April 23

Choices A, B, and D are incorrect because they do not represent the date calculated using Naegele's Rule.

2. The maternal health nurse is taking the intake history of a 26-year-old woman who is 5 months pregnant. She has several unexplained bruises on her arms, is avoiding eye contact with the nurse, and is replying to the nurse's assessment questions in a quiet voice, using only one-word answers. The nurse would provide careful observation for which common occurrence in pregnancy?

    A. Chronic depression
    B. Physiological anemia
    C. Domestic violence
    D. Acute Insomnia

Rationale:

Correct answer: C

The occurrence of domestic violence, unfortunately, increases while a woman is pregnant. Signs of domestic violence while pregnant include late onset of prenatal care, much like the patient discussed above, who is at her intake appointment in her 5th month of pregnancy. Unexplained bruising, social withdrawal, depression, difficulty adhering to prenatal care recommendations, frequent missed appointments, and substance abuse are other characteristic findings in pregnant patients experiencing domestic violence.

Choice A is incorrect. While some women may feel depressed while pregnant, chronic depression varies from pregnancy to pregnancy. Unexplained bruising is not an expected finding in a depressed patient.

Choice B is incorrect. The occurrence of physiological anemia does increase during pregnancy but is not associated with a late onset of prenatal care and does not present with social withdrawal and depression.

Choice D is incorrect. Insomnia does sometimes occur during pregnancy but is not related to unexplained bruising or late onset of prenatal care.

3. The nurse is evaluating her prenatal client for sexually transmitted infections by looking for risk factors. Which of the following are considered risks of acquiring an STI? Select all that apply.

  A. Low socioeconomic status
  B. A monogamous relationship
  C. A history of working in the sex industry

D. Illicit drug use

E. History of cancer

F. Previous history of STIs

Rationale:

Correct answer: A, C, D, F

Low socioeconomic status, a history of being a sex worker, illicit drug use, and a previous history of sexually transmitted infections are all risk factors for developing STIs while pregnant. Other factors include multiple sexual partners and being unmarried.

B and E are incorrect because a history of cancer and monogamous relationships are not examples of risk factors for acquiring an STI.

4. The prenatal client is 7 months pregnant and would like to start an exercise regimen. The nurse knows which of the following exercises is most appropriate at this point in her pregnancy?

A. Bike riding

B. Running

C. Zumba

D. Swimming

Rationale:

Correct answer: D

Swimming is the most appropriate workout at this point in the mother's pregnancy. Swimming is low impact and does not require balancing, which can be difficult with the excess weight a woman carries in her third trimester.

Choices A, B, and C are incorrect. These activities require careful balance and are too high impact for a woman who is just starting an exercise regimen. Generally, a cardiovascular exercise regimen should be established before the pregnancy begins.

5. The prenatal client asks the nurse when she might be able to find out the gender of her fetus. The most appropriate response by the nurse is:

    A. "The first ultrasound, done between 9-12 weeks, will be able to determine a viable fetal heartbeat as well as the gender."

    B. "An ultrasound done at weeks 13-14 can potentially detect fetal characteristics of Down Syndrome and can also confirm gender."

    C. "The routine ultrasound done at weeks 18-20 can detect gender and congenital malformations."

    D. A third trimester scan done near 30 weeks will determine the gender of your baby and will also reveal placental location."

Rationale:

Correct answer: C

The nurse would be most correct in informing the patient that she may know the gender of her baby between 18-20 weeks of pregnancy or at 5 months.

Choice A is incorrect. The first ultrasound is generally done between 9-12 weeks to detect fetal heartbeat, but gender is not yet visible by 2D ultrasound.

Choice B is incorrect because an ultrasound at weeks 13-14 can reveal characteristics of Down Syndrome but is too early to confirm gender.

Choice D is incorrect. Placental location can be revealed by a 30-week ultrasound, but gender is generally revealed by ultrasound earlier than 30 weeks.

6. The nurse reads the history of the patient who is 39 weeks pregnant and finds that she is experiencing "placenta previa." Knowing the circumstances surrounding this issue, the nurse knows not to perform which of the following common procedures?

    A. Ultrasonography of the abdomen
    B. Palpating the uterus to determine fetal presentation
    C. Checking the cervix for dilation
    D. Placing the patient on her left side

Rationale:

Correct answer: C

If the prenatal client has a current history of placenta previa, the cervix should not be checked for dilation. Placenta previa occurs when the placenta develops in an inconvenient spot, either very close or atop the cervical opening. To prevent bleeding or premature labor, women with placenta previa should not have their cervix checked by internal exam. Instead, an ultrasound may be ordered. If an internal vaginal exam is needed, it should be performed in the OR under sterile conditions. Symptoms of placenta previa include painless bright red bleeding. Complications include impaired fetal gas exchange and risk for fluid volume deficit.

Choice A is incorrect. Ultrasounds may be performed safely on women with placenta previa. In fact, ultrasounds are the best way to evaluate cervical dilation and confirm location of placenta in a woman with this issue.

Choice B is incorrect. If required by the physician, the nurse may palpate the abdomen of a woman whose pregnancy is complicated by placenta previa. Understanding fetal presentation may aid in delivery, which will likely be a C-section.

Choice D is incorrect. Laying on her left side is a safe position for pregnant women, including those with placenta previa. Laying on the left side increases circulation to the fetus and is often a comfortable position for laboring women. When diagnosed with placenta previa, the mother should be placed on bedrest initially for 72 hours, either in a side-lying position or in Trendelenburg position.

7. The obstetric nurse is looking over her laboring prenatal client's chart. When the nurse sees that her patient is suffering from pre-eclampsia, she knows to watch for which complications in the newborn fetus?

   A. Disseminated Intravascular Coagulation (DIC)
   B. Low birthweight
   C. Decreased liver enzymes
   D. Blurred vision

Rationale:

Correct answer: B

The nurse with this patient should be aware that the newborn may likely be born at a low birthweight. Because pre-eclampsia often results in blood being shunted away from the fetus, growth restriction is commonly found in infants born to these mothers.

Choice A is incorrect because DIC is a risk for the mother who is in severe eclampsia. This is not a likely risk to the fetus of a mother with pre-eclampsia.

Choice C is incorrect because mothers with pre-eclampsia are at risk for HELLP syndrome (hemolysis, elevated liver enzymes, low platelet count).

Choice D is incorrect because blurred vision is seen in mothers who are suffering from pre-eclampsia, not their infants.

8. The prenatal client has just arrived at the clinic and reports a period that is three days late and a positive home urine pregnancy test. She asks the nurse about the following assessments and procedures. The nurse would be correct in stating that which of these procedures would not be performed at this time?

   A. Calculation of body mass index (BMI)
   B. Pelvic examination
   C. Evaluation of areas prone to edema such as hands, feet, and face
   D. Fetal doppler

Rationale:

Correct answer: D

A fetal doppler would not be appropriate at this appointment. Because this patient is only three days late for her period, she is likely between 4 and 5 weeks pregnant which is too soon to hear fetal heart tones by doppler. Fetal heart tones will be heard by doppler at 8-12 weeks pregnant. Assessing by doppler at this time will cause unnecessary stress on the mother, because absent heart tones this early in a pregnancy are not a cause for concern.

Choice A is incorrect. Evaluating a pregnant patient's body mass index (BMI) is common practice at the start of the pregnancy. It serves as a base point for weight gain and will help the nurse establish the plan of care. Women who have a BMI less than 18.5 (underweight) should be encouraged to gain 18-40 lbs. during the pregnancy. A BMI of 18.5-24.9 (normal weight) requires 25-35 lbs. of weight gain during the pregnancy. BMI 25-29.9 (overweight) will be cautioned not to gain more than 15-25 lbs. during the pregnancy. And BMI 30 or over (obesity) should gain no more than 11-20 lbs. throughout the course of the pregnancy.

Choice B is incorrect. Pelvic examinations are routinely performed at the first prenatal check up for a pregnant client.

Choice C is incorrect. Ensuring that no edema is present and that the mother is not experiencing edema is common practice in the prenatal clinic. Many women experience mild swelling while pregnant, generally in the later months. Evaluating the patient's level of edema will serve as a baseline for the following months.

9. Diabetes affects some women more than others. Based on race, which of the following women are not at a heightened risk of developing gestational diabetes?

   A. Native American
   B. Japanese
   C. African American
   D. Hispanic

Rationale:

Correct answer: B

Of these races, Asian-American women are less likely to develop gestational diabetes than others. Other risk factors include obesity, family history of diabetes, personal history of gestational diabetes, hypertension, recurrent UTIs, polyhydramnios, and a previously large infant (greater than 9 lbs. or 4000 g).

Choices A, C, and D are incorrect. Native Americans, African Americans, Hispanics, and Polynesians are all at an increased risk for developing gestational diabetes while pregnant.

10. The prenatal client is believed to be about 6 weeks pregnant. Which of the following methods is the most accurate way to determine fetal gestational age?

   A. Naegele's Rule
   B. Fundal measurement
   C. Ultrasound
   D. HcG levels

Rationale:

Correct answer: C

When the patient is between 6 and 10 weeks pregnant, ultrasound (fetal head measurements) estimations of fetal age will be the most accurate. Accuracy decreases with growth of fetus when biological and environmental factors begin playing a role.

Choice A is incorrect. Naegele's Rule is used to calculate an estimated due date based on the last menstrual period but is not more accurate than an ultrasound.

Choice B is incorrect. At about 6 weeks, fundal measurement will be less reliable than an ultrasound. Fundal height does not reach above the level of the symphysis pubis until about 12-14 weeks pregnant.

Choice D is incorrect. HcG levels can vary widely from woman to woman. HcG is tested for, commonly, in urine and blood, with serum results being more sensitive. Increased HcG levels are a probable sign of pregnancy but are not an accurate way to determine the fetal gestational age.

11. The pregnant, 34-year-old client is discussing vaccines with the nurse. The client has a history of tuberculosis. Which of the following statements is best for the nurse to make when communication with this client?

    A. "You should receive your annual flu vaccine if you have not received it for this season."
    B. "If you have not had the chicken pox, you should consider getting your varicella vaccination."
    C. "Have you had the German measles? If not, we can schedule your immunization."
    D. "The human papilloma virus is dangerous while pregnant, so we should schedule your vaccination today."

Rationale:

Correct answer: A

The prenatal client should receive a flu vaccination if she's not yet had one for the current or upcoming flu season. Since the seasonal flu vaccine does not contain live viruses, it is safe and recommended in pregnancy.

Choice B is incorrect. The varicella vaccine is not recommended during pregnancy because it is a live virus. This vaccine may cause fetal scarring, microcephaly, limb atrophy, and other congenital abnormalities.

Choice C is incorrect. The German measles vaccination is generally given as a packaged vaccine as a component of the MMR vaccination. This vaccine may also cause congenital abnormalities as well as miscarriage.

Choice D is incorrect. The human papilloma virus vaccine is not safe to give to a prenatal client.

12. The prenatal client is being seen in the clinic for her first prenatal office visit. The nurse reads through the patient's chart and notices that she has a history of a blighted ovum. The nurse knows that a blighted ovum is most likely to occur at which point during pregnancy?

    A. 8-12 weeks
    B. 16-20
    C. 22-26
    D. 30-34

Rationale:

Correct answer: A

A blighted ovum (anembryonic pregnancy) occurs when the early fertilized egg implants in the uterus but doesn't develop into an embryo. The gestational sac is often left intact. Most cases of blighted ovum occur between 8 and 12 weeks. The cause is usually chromosomal abnormalities, and this is the cause of about 50% of first trimester miscarriages.

Choice B is incorrect because a blighted ovum usually occurs earlier than 16-20 weeks, before a woman even knows she is pregnant.

Choice C is incorrect because early ultrasound will detect lack of fetal heart tones with blighted ovum, and this often happens before 22-26 weeks.

Choice D is incorrect because blighted ovum cases generally occur during the first trimester or earlier than 12 weeks.

13. A prenatal patient has been hospitalized for symptomatic and worsening HELLP syndrome at 38 weeks' gestation. The nurse knows that which treatment will be of most help to prevent further complications of this dangerous condition?

    A. Immediate caesarean delivery of the fetus
    B. Intravenous fluid replacement with magnesium sulfate
    C. Routine blood pressure checks
    D. Strict bed rest

Rationale:

Correct answer: A

Mothers with severe pre-eclampsia (BP greater than 160/110 mmHg), often occurring in the later stages of pregnancy or even after childbirth, are at risk for HELLP syndrome (hemolysis, elevated liver enzymes, low platelet count). While immediate delivery of the fetus may not be necessary in a woman with asymptomatic HELLP syndrome, women over 37 weeks' gestation and with worsening symptoms are generally treated via delivery of the fetus. A caesarean section is generally planned.

Choice B is incorrect. While magnesium sulfate may be employed to prevent or treat seizures from prenatal hypertension or HELLP syndrome, it is not the most helpful implementation for this condition.

Choice C is incorrect. Women with HELLP syndrome should have routine vital sign checks, especially blood pressure readings. However, monitoring blood pressure regularly will not prevent further complications of HELLP syndrome (such as pulmonary edema, acute renal failure, liver failure and death) more than immediate delivery.

Choice D is incorrect. Strict bed rest may be initiated upon hospitalization, but it will not solve this client's serious condition or prevent the complications listed above. At 38 weeks' gestation, the woman is full-term, so the best way to protect her from deterioration is immediate delivery of the child.

14. The prenatal client is asking her nurse about physical changes during pregnancy. In her 20th week, she notices that her skin seems darker than normal. The nurse explains that this phenomenon is:

   A. Abnormal and should be addressed by a dermatologist; rare forms of skin cancer can occur during the second trimester.
   B. Abnormal and may need to be treated with intravenous fluids.
   C. Common and is a result of increased tissue perfusion.
   D. Expected and is caused by increased melanin production.

Rationale:

Correct answer: D

Pregnancy glow is a real phenomenon and is thought to be a result of an increase in melanin production. Pregnant women may experience blotchy brownish areas on the forehead and cheeks (chloasma or "mask of pregnancy"), darkening skin, and/or the development of a linea nigra (darkened vertical skin line extending from the symphysis pubis to the umbilicus).

Choice A is incorrect. Risk for rare skin cancers does not increase during pregnancy.

Choice B is incorrect. This condition is not abnormal and does not require treatment with intravenous fluids.

Choice C is incorrect because although these darkened skin changes are common and expected during pregnancy, the cause is not an increase in tissue perfusion.

15. Between the 16th and 20th weeks of pregnancy, a "multiple marker screening" or "quad screening" is performed via a blood draw in a laboratory or clinic. Which of the following statements by the nurse is not appropriate when communicating with the pregnant client about this test?

   A. "This test may be able to detect Down syndrome in your baby."
   B. "Although spina bifida is rare, it's a neural tube defect that we can look for with this test."
   C. "The quad screening will assess for cystic fibrosis in your fetus."
   D. "A rare chromosomal abnormality, aneuploidy, can be determined with this screening."

Rationale:

Correct answer: C

Cystic fibrosis (CF), a hereditary dysfunction of exocrine glands, which leads to thickened mucous production and altered pancreatic enzyme secretion, is generally determined after delivery, and not tested for with the quad screening. A sweat test done on the infant after delivery can lead to a CF diagnosis.

Choice A is incorrect. Quad screening tests for Down syndrome (extra chromosome number 21), so this is an appropriate statement for the nurse to make when talking with the pregnant client. Down syndrome is seen more commonly with maternal age greater than 35.

Choice B is incorrect. Spina bifida, a congenital anomaly of the spinal cord (nonunion between the laminae of the vertebrae) can be detected with a maternal quad test. This is an appropriate statement for the nurse to make. Mothers of advanced maternal age are also at greater risk for carrying a fetus with spina bifida.

Choice D is incorrect. Aneuploidy (altered chromosome numbers) is specifically looked for in prenatal clients undergoing a quad screening, so this is a correct statement.

16. The newly pregnant client is asking her nurse questions about typical tests ran during pregnancy. Which statement is most appropriate for the nurse to make when talking with the client?

    A. "Gestational diabetes can be determined at about 12 weeks' gestation."

    B. "A cardiac test at 16 weeks' gestation can determine cardiac disease, which may require additional specialized fetal monitoring during your labor and delivery."

    C. "A blood test at 32-36 weeks' gestation may alert your healthcare provider to a dangerous condition called abruptio placenta."

    D. "A glucose tolerance test will be conducted at about 24 weeks' gestation to check for gestational diabetes."

Rationale:

Correct answer: D

Most pregnant women are tested for gestational diabetes through a glucose testing procedure performed at about 6 months pregnant, or 24-28 weeks, so this is an appropriate statement for the nurse to make.

Choice A is incorrect because the glucose tolerance test is not routinely conducted this early in the pregnancy.

Choice B is incorrect because although cardiac disease during pregnancy does require additional fetal ` monitoring surrounding delivery, no specific blood test for cardiac disease is performed at 16 weeks' gestation.

Choice C is incorrect because abruptio placenta cannot be determined by a blood test. Symptoms include painful, dark red bleeding, painful and tender, tense abdomen, and the presence of uterine contractions. The risk for abruptio placenta is higher for mothers with a history of cocaine abuse or current hypertension.

17. To evaluate a fetus's risk of developing bacterial sepsis, bacterial pneumonia, or meningitis, the health care provider will generally order which exam at about 8 months' gestation?

    A. Multiple marker screening
    B. Group B strep
    C. HIV
    D. Syphilis

Rationale:

Correct answer: B

An active infection of Group beta streptococcus may cause deadly consequences in neonates. To prevent neonatal sepsis, pneumonia, or meningitis, the doctor will check the prenatal client for Group B strep at 8 months' gestation, and, if positive, treat with antibiotics (penicillin).

Choice A is incorrect because this is the quad screening, done between 15 and 20 weeks' gestation, which does not test for group B strep.

Choice C is incorrect because the HIV test is routinely performed at the first prenatal visit and sometimes repeated for high-risk clients in the third trimester.

Choice D is incorrect because pregnant clients are tested for syphilis at the first prenatal visit and rescreened in the third trimester if at high-risk.

18. The nurse is caring for a pregnant client whose fetus is suspected of suffering from intrauterine growth restriction. At 34 weeks pregnant, the health care provider has ordered non-stress tests to monitor the fetal well-being. The nurse knows that this monitoring should be discontinued at what point?

    A. When the patient has 3 reassuring results in a row
    B. When the patient is no longer symptomatic
    C. After delivery of the fetus
    D. Once symptoms worsen, and more aggressive methods should be implemented

Rationale:

Correct answer: C

In a patient whose fetus is suspected of having IUGR, or intrauterine growth restriction, non-stress tests should be continued until the infant is born.

Choice A is incorrect. Since non-stress tests are used to evaluate *current* fetal oxygenation rather than future fetal health, non-stress tests should be continued, even if results are reassuring.

Choice B is incorrect. Generally, the mother will not have symptoms other than a smaller than normal uterus if her fetus is suspected of suffering from IUGR.

Choice D is incorrect. More aggressive monitoring methods include scalp monitoring during labor so are not used in a non-laboring 34-week pregnant patient.

19. The prenatal client with cervical insufficiency is curious about when her cervical cerclage will be removed. The nurse would be most correct when providing this patient with which information?

    A. At the onset of labor
    B. Around 40 weeks' gestation
    C. 37 weeks' gestation
    D. Before the performance of a C-section

Rationale:

Correct answer: C

Surgical cerclage is a purse-string type suture used to treat an incompetent cervix, to allow a woman to make it to full-term in her pregnancy. Most health care providers will remove a woman's cervical cerclage at about 37 weeks' gestation. Before this point, the fetus has a greater risk of suffering from complications related to pre-term birth.

Choice A is incorrect. While a cervical cerclage will be removed if true labor is impending, this is not the best time to remove a cervical cerclage.

Choice B is incorrect. Most health care providers will attempt to remove a cervical cerclage before 40 weeks' gestation.

Choice D is incorrect. While a cerclage may be removed before a C-section, a cervical cerclage is generally removed in hopes of vaginal delivery.

20. The prenatal client is being prepared for a C-section. The nurse knows that the best position in which to place the patient while awaiting anesthesia is which of the following?

    A. Trendelenburg
    B. Semi-fowler's position

C. Supine with a pillow under the right hip

D. Supine with flexed knees

Rationale:

Correct answer: C

The best position to support maternal comfort and sufficient blood flow to both mother and fetus before a c-section is supine with a pillow under the right hip.

Choice A is incorrect because in Trendelenburg position, the patient is supine with the foot of the bed elevated 15-30 degrees. This position places the weight of the baby and the uterus on the diaphragm and may make it hard for the pregnant woman to breathe and may also impair venous return.

Choice B is incorrect because turning the woman on her side maximizes blood flow back to the heart.

Choice D is incorrect because this position does not facilitate easy breathing or blood flow in the pregnant client awaiting anesthesia for c-section.

21. The nurse is evaluating the post-partum client, still numb from her epidural, for the presence of hematoma. Which of the following would indicate the presence of this condition?

A. Complaints of stabbing pain

B. Vital sign changes

C. Complaints of skin tears

D. Signs of heavy bruising

Rationale:

Correct answer: B

Vital changes are the most accurate indicators of a developing hematoma.

Choices A and C are incorrect. Because this patient is still numb from her epidural, she is unlikely to feel these types of pain.

Choice D is incorrect. Signs of bruising may be present but may not be initially noticeable.

22. While assessing the post-natal client's abdomen, the nurse finds the uterus boggy and soft. Which of the following nursing actions takes the highest priority?

A. Reporting findings to the primary health care provider

B. Pushing against the uterus to expel tissue

C. Documenting the findings

D. Massaging the fundus until firm

Rationale:

Correct answer: D

The priority nursing intervention in a case of a soft and boggy uterus is to massage the uterus until firm.

Choice A is incorrect. If this condition continues, notifying the primary health care provider may be appropriate, but the nurse should focus on bedside nursing interventions that treat the specific problem ahead of calling the healthcare provider.

Choice B is incorrect. Pushing against the uterus could cause uterine injury or hemorrhage and will increase pain.

Choice C is incorrect. While documenting the findings is appropriate, it should not be completed until the uterus has been massaged. Direct patient care always takes priority over documentation.

23. The post-natal client has developed cystitis. What action should the nurse perform first?

    A. Monitoring hematocrit and hemoglobin levels
    B. Icing the patient's perineum
    C. Offering plenty of warm baths
    D. Encouraging plentiful fluid intake

Rationale:

Correct answer: D

Cystitis, or bladder infection, is best managed with plenty of fluids. Post-natal clients with cystitis should drink at least 3,000 mL of water daily.

Choice A is incorrect. While some blood loss may occur through the urine in cases of cystitis, lowered Hgb and Hct is not generally a concern.

Choice B is incorrect. Icing the perineum relieves pain from vaginal birth but does not relieve bladder discomfort or treat the infection associated with cystitis.

Choice C is incorrect. Warm baths are better suited for use in patients with perineal pain and do not treat the underlying cause of cystitis.

24. The labor and delivery nurse is evaluating her patient for a superficial venous thrombosis. Which of the following symptoms indicate the presences of an SVT?

    A. Paleness of the calf
    B. Cool calves
    C. Palpable dorsalis pedis pulses
    D. Hard and enlarged veins

Rationale:

Correct answer: D

Women experiencing a superficial venous thrombosis will present with hard and large veins.

Choice A and B are incorrect. Patients with SVTs will have warm and erythematic skin around the site, rather than pale and cool calves.

Choice C is incorrect. Palpable dorsalis pedis pulses are normal findings and not indicative of an SVT.

25. The clinic nurse is educating a prenatal client on the success rates of external cephalic version, or ECV. After discussing positive influences on the procedure, the nurse would recognize that this patient would be most likely to have a successful ECV if:

    A. The placenta is attached anteriorly.
    B. Her fetus is in a transverse position.
    C. She has an amniotic fluid index of 11.
    D. She has placenta previa.

Rationale:

Correct answer: B

Factors that positively influence the success of ECV include having a fetus in transverse lie or oblique lie, an amniotic fluid index below 10, and a posteriorly attached placenta. Women of Black heritage are also more likely to have a successful ECV procedure.

Choice A is incorrect because an anteriorly attached placenta can negatively impact the effectiveness of an ECV procedure.

Choice C is incorrect because an amniotic fluid index above 10 increases risks for complications with the ECV procedure.

Choice D is incorrect because an ECV procedure will not be performed on a mother with placenta previa.

26. The prenatal nurse is providing education to a newly pregnant mother about the growth of the uterus during pregnancy. She explains that the size of the uterus is often compared to fruit. During the fourth month of pregnancy, a woman often begins to "show," and her uterus is often compared to which of the following fruits?

    A. Grapefruit
    B. Plum
    C. Cantaloupe
    D. Apple

Rationale:

Correct answer: A

During the fourth month of pregnancy the uterus is generally compared to the size of a grapefruit. The fundal height will be palpable and located midway between the pubic symphysis and the navel.

Choice B is incorrect. The uterus is compared to a plum between 6 and 8 weeks of pregnancy.

Choice C and D are incorrect. These comparisons are generally not made once the uterus is noticeably palpable and easily measured.

27. The nurse is reading lab results before seeing her prenatal client. Noting that hCG levels were 4,000 mIU/mL 3 days before, the nurse will expect today's levels to be:

    A. 4,500 mIU/mL

    B. 13,000 mIU/mL

    C. 8,000 mIU/mL

    D. 5,000 mIU/mL

Rationale:

Correct answer: C

During the first trimester, hCG levels are expected to double every 2-3 days. This patient's hCG levels should be about 8,000 mIU/mL three days after the previous lab values were drawn.

Choices B, C, and D are incorrect because they do not reflect an hCG level that doubles within 2-3 days.

28. Which of the following herbal supplements, often taken for treating UTIs or cystitis, should the nurse warn the patient against taking because of its risk to the liver?

    A. Ginkgo biloba
    B. Uva ursi
    C. Acetaminophen
    D. Topical tea tree oil

Rationale:

Correct answer: B

Uva ursi, often used to improve bladder health, can cause liver damage, especially when taken for more than 5 days in a row. Because of this, pregnant women should not take uva ursi.

Choice A is incorrect. While it's true that pregnant women should avoid taking ginkgo biloba, this herbal supplement is used for memory function, not urinary health. Still, pregnant women should be warned against taking this supplement as it may cause hemorrhage.

Choice C is incorrect. Although acetaminophen may be hepatotoxic if taken in large doses, it is not an herbal supplement and may be used as directed by the woman's physician during pregnancy.

Choice D is incorrect. Topical tea tree oil is often used to relieve itching, and pain related to yeast infections and is safe to apply topically while pregnant.

29. The nurse is reviewing assigned patients for the shift. Out of these four women in labor, which patient's neonate is at the largest risk of developing hemolytic disease of the newborn?

    A. The mother with jaundice
    B. The mother with HIV
    C. The mother who is Rh negative
    D. The mother receiving antibiotics for Group B strep

Rationale:

Correct answer: C

Mothers who are Rh negative are at risk for delivering infants with hemolytic disease of the newborn. If the baby's blood type is Rh positive, the plasma of the mother's blood may create antibodies to attack the baby's D antigens. Since the blood type of the fetus is unknown until after birth, treatment for this dangerous disease includes plasma exchanges in the mother prior to delivery and maternal Rh immune globulin administration.

Choice A is incorrect. Hemolytic disease of the newborn causes jaundice in the newborn, not the mother.

Choice B is incorrect. An HIV mother can be treated during pregnancy to significantly decrease the risk of transmitting HIV to her baby. There is no link between an HIV mother and hemolytic disease of the newborn, unless the mother is Rh negative.

Choice D is incorrect because antibiotics do not cause hemolytic disease of the newborn.

30. The prenatal client is experiencing morning sickness but is concerned about the safety of certain herbal supplements and medications used to combat nausea. The nurse would be most correct in stating that which remedy for morning sickness is considered the safest?

    A. Calabash clay
    B. Ondansetron
    C. Ginger
    D. Metoclopramide

Rationale:

Correct answer: C

Out of these herbal and pharmaceutical options, ginger is the safest remedy for morning sickness. 250 mg ginger taken four times a day has been found to be effective for mild-to-moderate nausea and vomiting related to pregnancy (pregnant women should not exceed 1 g of ginger per day).

Choice A is incorrect. Calabash clay, also known as Nzu, is an African remedy for morning sickness. The FDA has warned against using this remedy, as it could possibly contain lead or arsenic, and can be harmful to both the mother and the fetus.

Choice B is incorrect. While Ondansetron is used during pregnancy for cases of morning sickness resulting in weight loss or failure to gain, no medications are without risk during pregnancy. Some studies do show an increase in birth defects when prescription antiemetics are used regularly throughout the pregnancy.

Choice D is incorrect because metoclopramide can have negative side effects such as restlessness, anxiety, drowsiness, and can cause extrapyramidal symptoms and dystonic reactions. A natural antiemetic is safer for use in pregnancy and has less side effects for the mother and the fetus.

31. The nurse caring for an HIV-positive pregnant client is answering questions about testing of the newborn after birth. The nurse knows that screening of her neonate for human immunodeficiency virus will first occur:

    A. At birth

B. 14 -21 days after birth

C. 30 days after birth

D. In utero via amniocentesis

Rationale:

Correct answer: B

All HIV-infected pregnant women should take HIV medications during the pregnancy to protect their own health and to reduce the likelihood of transmission to the baby. Risk for transmission can be decreased to 2% if proper care is taken and HIV medications are used throughout the pregnancy. Infants who were exposed in utero to HIV should be tested 14 to 21 days after birth and then again at 1 to 2 months and 4 to 6 weeks.

Choice A is incorrect because the baby is generally not tested at birth. The first test occurs 2-3 weeks after delivery.

Choice C is incorrect because the first infant HIV test will generally be completed prior to one month of age.

Choice D is incorrect because amniocentesis should be avoided in HIV pregnant women because this procedure increases risk for transmission of HIV to the fetus.

32. The maternal health clinic nurse is discussing the plan of care with a prenatal client with gestational diabetes.

Which of the following is most important for the nurse to include?

A. "You will need to fast for twelve hours prior to your monthly lab draw."
B. "Be sure to take your oral hypoglycemic medication exactly as prescribed daily."
C. "Be sure to consume the prescribed amount of food daily and eat your meals at the same times each day."
D. "Avoid exercise for the remainder of the pregnancy to ensure your blood glucose levels don't drop too low."

Rationale:

Correct answer: C

A balanced diet with consistent daily calorie intake is a necessary component of patient education for a client with gestational diabetes. Additionally, the nurse must teach the client about home glucose monitoring, insulin injection, and the potential need for increased insulin dosage as the baby grows throughout the pregnancy.

Choice A is incorrect because the client may not necessarily require monthly lab draws. Frequent monitoring of blood glucose at home is required.

Choice B is incorrect because oral hypoglycemic are contraindicated for use in pregnant clients as these medications are teratogenic to the fetus.

Choice D is incorrect because clients with gestational diabetes should exercise daily.

33. The purpose for asking a prenatal client about her history with rheumatic fever has the most to do with:

    A. Cardiac stress related to a possible valvular lesion.
    B. Preventing transmission of this teratogenic condition to her infant.
    C. Preparing to deliver preventative antibiotics during labor and post-delivery.
    D. Monitoring lung sounds for reoccurrence of the disorder.

Rationale:

Correct answer: A

Rheumatic fever is a rare complication after a patient has had a streptococcal tonsillitis infection. It can lead to rheumatic heart disease and can occur 10-20 years after the original illness. Rheumatic fever can cause the formation of valvular lesions which can lead to cardiac stress during pregnancy.

Choice B is incorrect because a prenatal client with a history of rheumatic fever will not be at risk for passing on rheumatic fever to her infant.

Choice C is incorrect. Preventative antibiotics are not used to treat rheumatic heart disease.

Choice D is incorrect. Lung sounds are not relevant to a woman with a history of rheumatic fever.

34. The nurse is talking with a 6 weeks' pregnant woman in the prenatal clinic. The client asks if she will be able to hear the heartbeat of the embryo at this time. The appropriate nursing response is that the client will:

    A. Be able to hear the heartbeat via doppler at this time, but the gender cannot be confirmed via ultrasound.
    B. Will not be able to hear the heartbeat between 14-16 weeks' gestation.
    C. Hear the fetal heart tones via doppler around 10-12 weeks' gestation.
    D. Be scheduled for an amniocentesis if the heart tones are not heard at this time.

Rationale:

Correct answer: C

Fetal heart tones are generally first heard around 10-12 weeks' gestation.

Choice A is incorrect. Fetal heart tones cannot be heard at 6 weeks' gestation, nor can gender be determined by ultrasound.

Choice B is incorrect because by 14-16 weeks' gestation, the fetal heart tones should be heard via doppler at each office visit.

Choice D is incorrect because at 6 weeks' gestation, the fetal heart tones are not expected to be heard. Lack of fetal heart tones at 6 weeks is not an indication for an amniocentesis at this time.

35. The nurse is providing preventative education to a group of pregnant women at the maternal health center. Which of the following statements regarding preeclampsia is inappropriate for the nurse to include in the patient education?

    A. "If your blood pressure is high at your first prenatal appointment, this is a condition called preeclampsia, which can be treated."
    B. "If you develop preeclampsia, it is often due to the kidneys malfunctioning, causing fluid overload."
    C. "If your blood pressure becomes elevated after 20 weeks' gestation, this is preeclampsia."
    D. "Caucasian women are at greater risk for preeclampsia than African American clients."

Rationale:

Correct answer: C

Pre-eclampsia occurs when a pregnant woman develops high blood pressure (greater than 140/90) after 20 weeks' gestation.

Choice A is incorrect. Elevated blood pressure which presents before 20 weeks is characterized as preexisting hypertension, unrelated to pregnancy.

Choice B is incorrect. Renal failure can be a result of eclampsia but is not the cause.

Choice D is incorrect because African American clients are at greater risk for developing pre-eclampsia than Caucasian clients.

36. A rubella infection of the pregnant mother can cause all of the following except for:

    A. Intrauterine growth restriction
    B. Hydrocephaly
    C. Large for gestational age infant
    D. Stillbirth

Rationale:

Correct answer: C

A rubella infection is not known for causing infants to be born large for their gestational age.

Choices A, B, and D are all possible complications in the infant born to a mother with a rubella infection.

37. Pregnancy increases a woman's risk of becoming a victim of domestic violence. Which following is not a symptom that requires further investigation into possible abuse?

    A. Depression
    B. Weight gain
    C. Unexplained bruising
    D. Late initiation of prenatal care

Rationale:

Correct answer: B

Weight gain is not a common symptom found in pregnant women who are victims of domestic violence. Risk for domestic violence is greater while a woman is pregnant. Signs include social withdrawal, difficulty adhering to prenatal care recommendations, frequent missed appointments, and substance abuse.

Choice A is incorrect because depression is commonly seen in pregnant women who are being abused.

Choice C is incorrect because unexplained bruises or injuries are a hallmark sign of domestic violence.

Choice D is incorrect because delayed initiation of prenatal care is often seen in women who are victim of domestic violence.

38. The estimated date of delivery method has been used for nearly 200 years and is performed by:

    A. Checking the length and color of the cervix.

    B. Counting 14-21 days from the first day of the last menstrual period.

    C. Counting 280 days forward from the first day of the woman's last menstrual period.

    D. Counting 246 days backwards from the date of conception.

Rationale:

Correct answer: C

The EDD method is performed by counting 280 days from the first day of a woman's last menstrual period.

Choice A is incorrect. Assessing a softened, bluish colored cervix is a probable sign of pregnancy and is known as Chadwick's sign. However, this assessment does not help to determine a woman's estimated due date.

Choice B is incorrect. This describes how the estimated date of conception is calculated.

Choice D is incorrect. Counting 246 days from the date of conception is irrelevant to determining EDD. Date of conception is often unknown, because it depends on the day of ovulation, which us usually unspecified.

39. The lab results have returned to the clinic on one of the nurse's prenatal clients. She is 8 weeks pregnant and has a hematocrit level of 32% and hemoglobin of 11.7. These numbers are decreased from her pre-pregnancy baseline levels. What is the next best action the nurse should take?

    A. Call the mother and ask that her levels be redrawn
    B. Record these normal findings in the client's medical record
    C. Report this abnormal finding to the healthcare provider immediately
    D. Call the mother and discuss prenatal vitamins and nutritional requirements during pregnancy

Rationale:

Correct answer: D

Normal hematocrit for a woman is 35-47%, and normal hemoglobin for a woman is 12-16 g/dL. These results are both slightly decreased, outside of the normal range.

While this is common during pregnancy due to the increased circulating blood volume, the safest nursing action is to educate the client about increasing iron in the diet and maintaining good nutrition throughout the remainder of her pregnancy.

Choice A is incorrect because there is no reason to believe the lab values are falsely low. The nurse should not assume that the levels need to be reassessed.

Choice B is incorrect because documentation is not more important than patient education about nutrition.

Choice C is incorrect because educating the patient is more important than notifying the healthcare provider. The values are slightly low, indicating anemia. This is not a medical emergency that requires the healthcare provider right now.

40. A new mother has just given birth to an infant with congenital abnormalities related to a maternal varicella infection in the first trimester of the pregnancy. The nurse knows that which is true about this newborn baby?

    A. The newborn a 30% mortality rate in the first four years of life
    B. The newborn has a high chance of being infected with neonatal chickenpox

C. May develop more severe symptoms of Congenital Varicella Syndrome in the next 3-60 days of life

D. The newborn cannot be breastfed

Rationale:

Correct answer: A.

A child born with congenital varicella syndrome (CVS) has a 30% mortality rate in the first four years of life.

Choice B is incorrect because if the mother's varicella infection was in the first trimester, the fetus would have received antibodies in utero to help fight the virus. Neonatal chickenpox is only seen in cases where the mother's varicella infection was near the end of the pregnancy, in which case the baby may not have received the antibodies in utero.

Choice C is incorrect because the symptoms of CVS are apparent at birth. The symptoms result from damage to the central nervous system during early fetal development. (They do not develop later in the baby's life.)

Choice D is untrue. A newborn with CVS will benefit from breastfeeding because the mother's breastmilk contains many necessary antibodies to help fight other diseases.

41. What does the term "nulligravida" describe?

A. A woman currently using birth control to avoid pregnancy

B. A woman who has never had any children

C. A woman who has had more than two previous live births

D. A woman prone to spontaneous abortions

Rationale:

Correct answer: B

Nulligravida refers to a woman who has never been pregnant.

Choice A is incorrect. Use of birth control does not indicate whether a woman has ever been pregnant in the past.

Choice C is incorrect. A woman who has had multiple children is considered to be multigravida.

Choice D is incorrect. A woman prone to spontaneous abortions has been pregnant, and thus is not nulligravida.

42. Chadwick's sign is a prenatal assessment performed at the initial clinic visit to verify pregnancy. Chadwick's sign presents as:

A. A blue to purplish hue to the cervix.

B. Softness to the uterine fundus felt through the abdomen.

C. A thinning and shortening of the cervix.

D. The absence of menstruation at day 28 in a woman's cycle.

Rationale:

Correct answer: A

Chadwick's sign presents as a blue to purple hue to the cervix.

Choice B is incorrect. A soft uterus is not used to verify pregnancy.

Choice C is incorrect. The thinning and shortening of the cervix is known as effacement and occurs just before or during labor.

Choice D is incorrect. The absence of menstruation is a subjective finding reported by the client and does not give any objective assessment data about the appearance of the cervix.

43. The 8-to-10-week ultrasound verifies all of the following except:

A. Estimated due date

B. Pelvic shape

C. The absence of fetal abnormalities

D. Confirmation of pelvic health

Rationale:

Correct answer: C

At the 8-to-10-week ultrasound, the radiologist will not be able to rule out all fetal abnormalities.

Choices A, B, and D are incorrect. Ultrasounds performed during this time period do help determine the due date as well as verify the pelvic shape and health.

44. A pregnant client expresses the desire to have freedom of movement and a drug-free labor and delivery, but she says she is not comfortable with a home birth. How should the nurse respond?

   A. "It is recommended that you deliver at the nearest hospital to your home."

   B. "A birthing center may be a good choice for you."

   C. "A home birth really may be best to meet your wishes."

   D. "Perhaps we can see if you can deliver in your clinician's office."

Rationale:

Correct answer: B

Benefits of a birthing center include more freedom to move around during labor, less medical intervention, more support for a drug-free labor, less likelihood of having an IV inserted, and more freedom to eat and drink during labor, if the mother chooses.

Choice A is incorrect. The nearest hospital may not be the best location for a pregnant woman concerned about her freedom of movement and a drug-free labor.

Choice C is incorrect. A woman who expresses she is not comfortable with a home birth should not be persuaded to have one. A home birth is more successful when the woman is confident about her birth choice.

Choice D is incorrect. Most deliveries do not occur at a clinician's office unless an emergency requires such.

45. Both the estimated date of delivery and Naegele's Rule are limited by the fact that they assume:

    A. Ovulation occurs on day 14 of a woman's menstrual cycle.
    B. Pregnancy lasts 9 months.
    C. Amenorrhea is the first sign of pregnancy.
    D. Women's menstrual cycles are 30 days in length.

Rationale:

Correct answer: A

Both EDD and Naegele's Rule are limited because they both assume that all women ovulate around 14 days into their menstrual cycle. Women's cycles all can vary biologically, and different clients may ovulate on varying days within their cycle. Estimated date of delivery can only be accurate if the estimated date of conception is accurate.

Choice B, C, and D are incorrect because they are not necessarily assumed with either EDD or Naegele's Rule.

46. A prenatal client at her fourth month clinic visit mentions that she has a tooth extraction procedure planned for the following month and is wondering whether or not she can continue with the procedure. With what information should the nurse provide the prenatal client?

   A. "There is no evidence that delaying dental health treatment in necessary during pregnancy."
   B. "You should wait until after delivery to have the procedure performed."
   C. "This procedure would be better performed in the third trimester."
   D. "Anti-viral medications should be taken before the procedure to prevent illness."

   Rationale:

Correct answer: A

There is no evidence that a pregnant woman will need to delay dental health treatment during pregnancy.

Choice B is incorrect. Waiting until after delivery is not required for a pregnant client to have routine dental work completed.

Choice C is incorrect. There is no reason to wait until the third trimester to perform this treatment.

Choice D is incorrect. Anti-viral medications should not be given to a pregnant woman who will be undergoing a dental procedure.

47. Using Naegele's Rule, what would a pregnant woman's estimated due date be if the first day of her last menstrual period was August 13?

    A. August 6 of the following year
    B. May 13 of the following year
    C. May 20 of the following year
    D. May 6 of the following year

Rationale:

Correct answer: C

Naegele's Rule requires the nurse to subtract three months from the first day of the client's last menstrual period, and then add seven days and one year. This woman would be due on May 20.

Choices A, B, and D are incorrect, according to Naegele's Rule for calculating a pregnant client's estimated date of delivery.

48. Which of the following issues does not correlate with an above-normal BMI pre-pregnancy?

    A. Gestational diabetes
    B. Pre-eclampsia
    C. Swelling
    D. Frequent UTI

Rationale:

Correct answer: D

Frequent UTIs do not correlate with above normal BMIs before pregnancy.

Choices A, B, and C are incorrect. Gestational diabetes, preeclampsia, and swelling are all associated with pre-pregnancy above normal BMI.

CHAPTER 3:

NCLEX-RN – MATERNITY: LABOR & BIRTH – POSTPARTUM - 25 QUESTIONS

1. The nurse caring for a patient in active labor would identify which of the following as examples of critical factors related to labor and birth? Select all that apply.

   A. Maternal pelvis
   B. Fetal attitude
   C. Previous birth experience
   D. Braxton-Hicks contractions
   E. Vulvar varicose veins

Rationale:

Correct answer: A, B, C

Five factors that play a critical role in labor and birth are: the passageway (which includes the size and type of the maternal pelvis) the passenger (including the fetal attitude, which is the flexion/extension of the fetal body and extremities), psychosocial considerations (such as previous birth experience) physiologic forces (such as the frequency, duration and intensity of active labor contractions) and position of the woman.

D is incorrect because Braxton-Hicks contractions, also known as prodromal labor, practice contractions, or false labor, are sporadic, infrequent, and irregular uterine contractions that sometimes start around six weeks' gestation but may not be felt until the second trimester. They do not play a critical role in labor and birth.

E is incorrect because the presence of varicose veins does not directly impact the labor and birth process. Vulvar varicose veins can occur during pregnancy as a result of the increased volume of blood circulating through the body and decreased rate of venous blood return back to the heart from lower extremities. Vulvar varicosities are often asymptomatic; however, they can cause discomfort during pregnancy. They usually disappear after birth and do not require treatment.

2. When admitting a patient to the birth center, the nurse notes that the woman has a platypelloid type pelvis. Which of the following is/are most likely to occur? Select all that apply.

    A. Fetal head must engage in the transverse position
    B. Normal vaginal delivery is likely

C. Delay of progress at the pelvic outlet

D. Arrest of labor

E. Risk for postpartum hemorrhage is decreased

Rationale:

Correct answer: A, C

With a platypelloid pelvis, the pelvic inlet is oval in shape with long transverse diameters. The pelvic outlet capacity is inadequate. As a result, when the fetal head engages, descent through the midpelvis can be difficult, and the progress of labor is delayed at the pelvic outlet. LOT position is critical for delivery through this pelvis type. Only about 3-5% of women have a platypelloid-shaped pelvis, and usually have difficulty delivering vaginally. Gynecoid and anthropoid type pelvises are considered favorable for normal vaginal birth.

B is incorrect because vaginal delivery can be quite difficult with this pelvis type. If the baby does not get into the appropriate LOT position, a caesarean delivery may be necessary.

D is incorrect because this shape of pelvis can prolong labor and make it difficult for the baby's head to engage but does not cause arrest of labor.

E is incorrect because this pelvis type can cause prolonged labor, which increases risk for bleeding. Postpartum hemorrhage risk is also increased with multiparity and retained placental fragments.

3. The nurse caring for a laboring woman determines that the fetal head is partially flexed, presenting the occipitofrontal diameter of the head, with the top of the head as the presenting part. Which is the most likely outcome?

    A. A normal vaginal birth
    B. The need to apply forceps to assist birth
    C. A cesarean birth
    D. The need to perform an external cephalic version

Rationale:

Correct answer: A

The information provided describes a sinciput/cephalic fetal presentation, which is usually transient, and as labor progresses, often converts to a vertex presentation. With conversion to vertex, the smallest diameter of the fetal head is presenting, facilitating a normal vaginal birth.

B is incorrect because use of forceps or vacuum extraction is not generally required when the baby's presentation is cephalic.

C is incorrect because this fetal presentation is ideal and does not often lead to a caesarean delivery.

D is incorrect because external cephalic version is performed to turn a fetus from a breech position or transverse position into a vertex position before labor begins.

4. A woman in preterm labor is given indomethacin to halt the labor. This medication is consistent with which possible cause of the onset of labor?

   A. Progesterone withdrawal
   B. Prostaglandin production
   C. Increased corticotropin-releasing hormone (CRH) levels
   D. Decreased levels of estrogen

Rationale:

Correct answer: B

Indomethacin is an NSAID, tocolytic medication which can delay birth for several days. The woman's body releases prostaglandins during labor, similar to the inflammatory response. The indomethacin suppresses the release of those prostaglandins, often stopping preterm labor. (Labor can be induced with vaginal application of prostaglandin E and reduced by suppressing prostaglandin production.)

A is incorrect because progesterone withdrawal is thought to play a role in the onset of labor, but the effectiveness of indomethacin is not related to progesterone.

C is incorrect because increased CRH levels are also unrelated to the use of indomethacin.

D is incorrect because increased estrogen levels, rather than decreased levels, are known to stimulate uterine muscle contractions to allow softening, stretching and thinning of the cervix.

5. A woman at 38 weeks' gestation has called the nurse to determine whether she should come to the birth center. She reports the appearance of bloody show and experiencing more intense uterine contractions. Which statement(s) by the mother indicates that she is experiencing false labor?

   A. "The pain begins in back and then comes around to my abdomen."
   B. "When I rest, the contractions are less intense."
   C. "The contractions are lasting longer each time."
   D. "Walking makes the contractions more intense."

Rationale:

Correct answer: B

False labor is characterized by irregular contractions that are not increasing in frequency, duration or intensity, and that will become less intense with walking, resting or a warm bath. The discomfort is usually centered in the abdomen, rather than beginning in back.

A is incorrect because this describes the pain associated with true labor contractions.

C is incorrect because increase in duration of contraction is a sign that labor is progressing.

D is incorrect because when activity strengthens contraction intensity it is a sign labor is progressing.

6. A woman at 40 weeks' gestation has come to the emergency department reporting moderately intense uterine contractions. Which signs indicate that the patient should be transferred to the labor and birth unit?

   A. Cervical dilation on admission at 3 cm, then at 5 cm 2 hours later
   B. The loss of a mucus plug in the woman's sanitary pad, with pink-tinged secretions
   C. The contractions are described as a feeling of "balling up" in the groin
   D. The cervix is firm and about 4 cm long

Rationale:

Correct answer: A

Progressive dilation and effacement of the cervix, as well as cervical softening, indicate the woman is in true labor, and cervical dilation of 4-7 cm indicates the active phase of labor, so the woman should be transferred to the labor and birth unit.

B is incorrect because loss of the mucus plug indicates that labor will typically occur within 24-48 hours, but the woman does not need to be admitted to the labor and birth unit at this time.

C is incorrect because regularity and intensity of contractions need to be assessed before determining if the woman is ready to be admitted for delivery.

D is incorrect because at the beginning of pregnancy, the cervix is firm and rigid, and about 3.5-4 cm in length. During labor, the cervix will thin and shorten in length.

7. The nurse caring for a woman during the second stage of labor understands that the cardinal movements of labor occur in which order? All options must be used.

    A. The fetal head is flexed so the chin moves onto the chest

    B. The fetal head moves downward toward the pelvic inlet

C. The fetal head passes beneath the symphysis pubis while in flexion

D. The fetal head rotates to fit the diameter of the pelvic cavity

E. The fetal shoulders rotate internally to fit the pelvis

F. The anterior, then posterior fetal shoulder passes under the symphysis pubis

Rationale:

Correct answer: B, A, D, C, E, F

The cardinal movements of labor occur in this order:

B - Descent - movement of the fetal head downwards until it reaches the pelvic inlet.

A - Flexion - when the fetal head reaches the pelvic floor, it then flexes so that the chin moves onto the chest, presenting the smallest anteroposterior diameter.

D - Internal rotation - The fetal head rotates from left to right, to fit the diameter of the pelvic cavity.

C - Extension - When internal rotation is complete, the fetal head passes beneath the synthesis pubis while in flexion.

E - External rotation - allows the fetal shoulders to rotate internally to fit the pelvis.

F - Expulsion - occurs as first the anterior, then the posterior fetal shoulder passes under the symphysis pubis.

8. The nurse caring for a woman in labor is preparing to determine the fetal position by palpation. Arrange the following maneuvers in the order the nurse should perform them. All options must be used.

   A. While facing the woman, the nurse palpates the right and left sides of the patient's abdomen using deep, but gentle, pressure.
   B. With the thumb and fingers of the right hand, the nurse gently grasps the lower portion of the abdomen just above the symphysis pubis.
   C. While facing the woman, the nurse palpates the upper abdomen with both hands.
   D. While facing the woman's feet, the nurse gently moves the fingers of both hands down the sides of the uterus towards the symphysis pubis.

Rationale:

Correct answer: C, A, B, D

Leopold's maneuvers are a systematic approach to evaluate the maternal abdomen and determine fetal position. The steps are:

C - Maneuver One: Fundal Grip - While facing the patient, the nurse should use both hands to palpate the upper abdomen to determine the shape, size, mobility, and consistence of what he or she feels. The nurse should feel that the limbs and shoulders contain little bone processes that move with the fetus's trunk; the head is firm, hard, round and moves separately from the trunk; and the buttocks is symmetric and feels soft.

A - Maneuver Two: Umbilical Grip - While still facing the patient, the nurse should next apply deep pressure with the palm of the hands to palpate the abdomen gently in order to identify the location of the fetus's back. This maneuver is performed by placing the right hand on one side of the patient's abdomen while using the left hand to explore the woman's uterus on the right side. Repeat this step on the opposite side using the opposite hand. The nurse should observe that the fetal back is smooth and firm. The extremities of the fetus should feel like protrusions and small irregularities. The back should connect with the form felt in the lower and upper abdomen.

B - Maneuver Three: Pawlick's Grip - During this step of the process, the nurse must identify the part of the fetus that is above the inlet, using the fingers and thumb of the right hand to grasp the lower abdominal area located above the pubic symphysis. The findings should validate what is determined in the first maneuver.

D - Maneuver Four: Pelvic Grip - This step of the process involves locating the fetus's brow. While facing the patient's feet, the nurse should gently move the fingers of both hands toward the pubis by sliding the hands over the sides of the patient's uterus. The side where there is greatest resistance to the descending fingers is the location of the brow. A well-flexed fetal head is located on the opposite side of the fetal back. If the head is extended, the back of the head is felt on the side where the back is located.

9. The nurse is providing care for a laboring woman and observes a drop in the fetal heart rate of more than 15 beats per minute. The decelerations occur near the beginning of the contraction and sometimes towards the peak of the contraction. The lowest fetal heart rate is reached in 20 seconds, and the duration of each deceleration is 45 seconds. Which of the following is the most likely cause for this fetal monitoring pattern?

   A. Autonomic nervous system stimulation caused by fetal head compression.
   B. Decreased oxygen transfer to the fetus.
   C. Environmental stimuli such as an internal vaginal exam

D. Vagal nerve stimulation related to compression of the umbilical cord.

Rationale:

Correct answer: D

The information provided describes variable decelerations, which are typically associated with vagal nerve stimulation related to umbilical cord compression during uterine contractions. This type of deceleration is usually not concerning and is considered normal if occurring before delivery and if accelerations are noted as well.

A is incorrect because autonomic nervous system stimulation related to fetal head compression results in FHR accelerations. This is a reassuring sign, signaling that the fetus is receiving adequate oxygen supply.

B is incorrect because late decelerations (occurring after the apex of the contraction) are an indication of fetal hypoxia.

C is incorrect because environmental stimuli, such as vaginal exams, can cause an episodic or periodic deceleration of the FHR that is not associated with uterine contractions.

10. The nurse providing care for a woman in active labor observes a pattern of fetal heart rate (FHR) decelerations characterized by an abrupt drop in FHR that shows as a jagged V shape on the monitor strip. The decelerations are not consistent in relation to the contractions. Which of these actions should be taken first?

    A. Administer 100% oxygen
    B. Administer oxytocin
    C. Check for cord prolapse
    D. Change position, possibly to Trendelenburg

Rationale:

Correct answer: D

The information provided refers to a fetal monitor pattern of variable decelerations. The first step is to reposition the woman in attempts to relieve cord compression and observe for FHR pattern improvement. If a position change is not effective, other nursing interventions may be needed.

A is incorrect because the woman's position should be changed before applying oxygen.

B is incorrect because if oxytocin is infusing and the variable decelerations continue after the woman's position has been changed, discontinuing the oxytocin is appropriate.

C is incorrect because the nurse should change the woman's position first and determine if the FHR pattern improves before performing a vaginal exam to check for cord prolapse.

11. The nurse providing care for a woman in labor observes a gradual decrease in fetal heart rate (FHR). The onset of the deceleration occurs at the peak of the contraction and slowly returns to baseline after the contraction is over. The time from onset to lowest point is 45 seconds. Which action should be taken first?

   A. Place the patient in a left-side-lying position
   B. Prepare oxytocin infusion
   C. Decrease intravenous fluid infusion to prevent fluid volume overload
   D. Prepare to assist the physician with fetal blood sampling

Rationale:

Correct answer: A

The information provided describes a fetal monitoring pattern of late decelerations, indicating uteroplacental insufficiency causing fetal hypoxia. The first nursing intervention that should be performed is to reposition the patient in a left-side-lying position and then administer oxygen at 7-10 L/min via face mask. The nurse should also provide the laboring woman with information about the FHR pattern and the interventions that will help.

B is incorrect because oxytocin should not be given when late decelerations are present.

C is incorrect because the IV fluid rate should be maintained or increased to maintain fluid volume and circulation for both the mother and the baby.

D is incorrect because fetal blood sampling is not the nurse's first priority when late.

12. While admitting a woman to the birthing center, the nurse notes that the patient is experiencing painless vaginal bleeding, with bright-red blood seen on the pad. The nurse's immediate actions include all of the following, with which exception?

    A. Assess fetal heart rate
    B. Notify healthcare provider immediately
    C. Perform vaginal examination
    D. Estimate amount of blood loss

Rationale:

Correct answer: C

Painless, bright red vaginal bleeding is a cardinal sign of placenta previa, where the placenta has implanted in the lower portion of the uterus near the internal cervical os. Vaginal examinations must be avoided because stimulation of the placenta may cause further hemorrhage.

A is incorrect because assessing the FHR is an appropriate nursing action when placenta previa is suspected. Non-reassuring fetal heart rate patterns should be reported right away.

B is incorrect because the healthcare provider should be immediately notified concerning significant bleeding.

D is incorrect because this is an appropriate nursing action. The nurse can weigh per-pads to determine blood loss volume. 1 gram = 1 mL of blood loss. It is important to monitor amount of bleeding very carefully, as changes in vital signs may not be evident, initially.

13. A woman in the first stage of labor has assumed a sitting position, leaning forward with the over-bed table for support. Which of the following describes a potential disadvantage of this position for labor?

    A. Back pain may be intensified
    B. Continuous fetal monitoring is not feasible
    C. Delays fetal descent
    D. May increase suprapubic discomfort

Rationale:

Correct answer: D

Sitting positions for labor may cause suprapubic pressure and increased discomfort.

A is incorrect because assuming a sitting position, leaning forward with support, will reduce back pain, as the fetus falls forward, away from the sacral promontory.

B is incorrect because this position will not interfere with continuous fetal monitoring.

C is incorrect because a sitting position enhances fetal descent due to gravity.

14. The certified nurse-midwife is caring for a woman in the second stage of labor and assists the woman to a seated position using a birthing stool. Which of the following are advantages of this position? Select all that apply.

    A. Improves fetal rotation
    B. Aids descent and expulsion of the infant.
    C. The woman is able to view the birth process
    D. Facilitates birth in the case of shoulder dystocia
    E. Faster episiotomy healing time

Rationale:

Correct answers: B, C

Advantages of a position sitting upright using a birthing stool are enhanced descent and expulsion of the infant due to gravity, and it allows the woman to view the birth of the infant. In addition, this position will not interfere with venous return from the lower extremities.

A is incorrect because if the nurse's goal is to rotate the fetus, this can be achieved by placing the woman on her hands and knees.

D is incorrect because a birthing stool does not facilitation birth in the case of shoulder dystocia (hands and knees position is better for shoulder dystocia).

E is incorrect because the birthing stool reduces the need for an episiotomy but does not directly facilitate perineal healing after delivery.

15. The nurse is caring for a woman in labor who has become restless and increasingly apprehensive and irritable. The nurse recognizes that these behaviors/symptoms are related to what?

    A. Phase 1 of the first stage of labor
    B. The fourth stage of labor
    C. The last phase of the first stage of labor
    D. Phase 2 of the second stage of labor

Rationale:

Correct answer: C

In the last phase of the first stage of labor, the transition phase, the laboring woman may become restless, frequently changing position. She is acutely aware of the increasing intensity of uterine contractions and may become more apprehensive and quite irritable.

A is incorrect because this is the latent phase of the first stage of labor in which dilation is measured at 0-3 cm and contractions are mild to moderate. Restlessness and acute discomfort are not common during this latent phase of stage 1.

B is incorrect because the fourth stage is the 4 hours after the placenta has been delivered, and the woman usually feels a huge sense of relief during this time period. She may sleep intermittently while also bonding with the baby.

D is incorrect because with the onset of the second stage of labor, the woman may feel a sense of relief that the birth is near, and regain a sense of control, especially if she is childbirth-prepared. She may sense an urgency to bear down, but the restlessness and irritability have usually subsided.

16. A first-time mother undergoing induction of labor with an oxytocin drip has experienced more than 6 contractions

over a period of 10 minutes. A vaginal exam reveals no progression of cervical effacement or dilation since the previous assessment. Fetal heart patterns are normal. Which actions by the nurse would represent appropriate care of this client? Select all that apply.

A. Assist the woman to a lateral position
B. Administer an intravenous bolus of 500 mL lactated Ringer's solution
C. Decrease oxytocin
D. Administer oxygen at 10 L/min via non-rebreather facemask
E. Encourage the woman to ambulate around the room

Rationale:

Correct answer: A, B, C

The information provided describes hypertonic contractions that are occurring more frequently than every 2 minutes, so the induction must be slowed. Nursing care management related to this labor pattern includes assisting the woman to a side-lying position and intravenous administration of a bolus of 500 mL of lactated Ringer's solution. The rate of the oxytocin drip should be decreased by at least half.

D is incorrect. Since the fetal heart rate pattern is normal, administration of oxygen is not indicated.

E is incorrect because ambulation will likely increase the frequency of contractions, so the nurse should encourage the woman to remain in bed and rest.

17. A gravida 5, para 4 woman is in active labor. Uterine contractions have decreased in frequency and intensity, with less than 3 contractions over a 10-minute period. Vaginal examination reveals that there has been no change in cervical dilation and effacement since the previous examination 2 hours before. Which of the following is the leading cause of this labor pattern?

    A. Fetal macrosomia
    B. Multiple gestation
    C. Malpresentation
    D. Hydramnios

Rationale:

Correct answer: A

The information provided describes a hypotonic labor pattern. Fetal macrosomia (excessive birth weight) occurs in one fourth of all pregnancies and is the leading cause of hypotonic labor. Other causes include sedation and cephalopelvic disproportion.

B, C, and D are incorrect because multiple gestation, malpresentation, and hydramnios are less common causes of hypotonic labor.

18. When assessing a woman 24 hours after giving birth, the nurse notes that the uterine fundus is deviated toward the right and is 1 finger breadth above the previous assessment. Which of the following immediate actions by the nurse would represent appropriate care of this client?

    A. Assess lochia for amount, color, odor, and clots
    B. Have the woman empty her bladder, then reassess
    C. Notify the physician or certified nurse-midwife
    D. Perform gentle massage of the uterine fundus

Rationale:

Correct answer: B

When assessment of the uterus reveals that the uterus is higher than expected and deviated to one side, distention of the bladder should be suspected. The nurse should have the woman empty her bladder, then reassess the uterus. If the woman is unable to void, it may be necessary to perform straight catheterization.

A is incorrect because assessment of lochia is part of postpartum assessment related to uterine involution, but with the findings described, the immediate action is to have the woman empty her bladder.

C is incorrect because immediate notification of the physician or certified nurse-midwife is not indicated until further nursing assessment has been made.

D is incorrect because gentle massage of the uterine fundus would be indicated if the uterus is boggy, indicating uterine atony.

19. The nurse is caring for a woman who gave birth the previous day and had previously expressed a desire to breastfeed her baby. She has been nursing the baby every 3-4 hours. Assessment of the breasts reveals a reddened area on one breast that is tender and warm to the touch. Which intervention should be included in the plan of care?

   A. Breastfeed the infant 8 -12 times every 24 hours from both breasts
   B. Breastfeed the infant every 2-3 hours from the unaffected breast only
   C. Bottle feed the infant using expressed breast milk
   D. Bottle feed the infant using infant formula

Rationale:

Correct answer: A

The assessment findings are consistent with mastitis, or inflammation of the breast. It is most commonly associated with backed up milk in one section of the breast. The woman should continue to breastfeed 8-12 times every 24 hours from both breasts. Discontinuation of breastfeeding will impact milk supply and does not honor the mother's desire to breastfeed. Current practice has shown that a breast infection resolves faster when breast engorgement is avoided and the risk of developing an abscess is decreased. For the baby, antibodies in the mother's milk protect the baby from bacteria associated with the infection. In almost all cases, the best intervention for a mother with mastitis is to keep nursing.

B is incorrect because even in the presence of infection, the woman can continue to breastfeed. In order to facilitate healing and develop adequate milk supply, she should nurse from both breasts.

C is incorrect because there is no need to offer milk from a bottle.

D is incorrect because it does not honor the woman's choice to breastfeed.

20. The nurse is providing postpartum care for a woman who has chosen not to breastfeed. Which information should be included in a teaching plan for this patient? Select all that apply.

A. The breasts should be firmly bound using elastic bandages

B. Bromocriptine will be prescribed to suppress milk production

C. Cold cabbage leaves will decrease local pain and swelling

D. Warm showers will reduce pressure by inducing leakage of milk

E. A well-fitting support bra will provide the needed support.

Rationale:

Correct answer: C, D, E

Measures to provide comfort for the woman who is not breastfeeding, or when weaning from the breast, include: application of cool cabbage leaves or ice packs inside the bra will help reduce pain and swelling; warm showers will induce milk leakage and help to relieve pressure related to engorgement; and a well-fitting support bra is needed to provide needed support.

A is incorrect because research findings show that women with bound breasts had more leakage, more pain, and needed more pain medication, compared to women using a supportive bra.

B is incorrect because pharmacological interventions such as bromocriptine were found to have untoward side effects such as myocardial infarction, cerebral angiopathy and thromboembolism, and have been taken off the market for milk cessation in the U.S.

21. The nurse is caring for a woman in the mother-baby care unit. Which intervention to relieve perineal pain is appropriate during the first 24 hours after giving birth? Select all that apply.

    A. Application of an ice pack
    B. A warm sitz bath
    C. Application of a warm compress
    D. A cool sitz bath
    E. PRN morphine

Rationale:

Correct answers: A, D

To help relieve perineal pain during the first 24 hours, the application of cold, including ice packs or cool sitz baths, will help reduce swelling and irritation.

B and C are incorrect because warmth is not used until after the first 24 hours.

E is incorrect because acetaminophen is the best drug for relieving perineal pain. Morphine is not commonly used.

22. The nurse has reviewed discharge instructions with a new mother who is breastfeeding her infant. Which statement, if made by the patient, would indicate a need for further discussion?

    A. When menstruation returns, I could get pregnant again.

    B. I can expect my period to return in about 12 weeks.

    C. My partner and I should abstain from intercourse until the lochia flow has stopped.

    D. I may experience vaginal dryness while I am breastfeeding.

Rationale:

Correct answer: A

While, for the breastfeeding woman, menstruation does not return until about 12 weeks or more after giving birth, it is important to remember that ovulation will occur prior to menses. Therefore, some birth control measure, such as a barrier method, may need to be used by the breastfeeding woman to prevent undesired pregnancies.

B is incorrect because it is a true statement; menstruation may not return until about 12 weeks or more after giving birth.

C is incorrect because current guidelines advise couples to abstain from intercourse until lochia flow has stopped and the episiotomy has healed, usually by 3 - 6 weeks postpartum.

D is incorrect because it is a true statement which indicates understanding of the instructions. As breastfeeding suppresses estrogen levels, the mother may experience vaginal dryness.

23. A student nurse is preparing to assess the perineum of a woman who has had an episiotomy. Which of the following nursing acronyms represents guidelines for performing this assessment?

   A. BUBBLE-LE
   B. REEDA
   C. HELLP
   D. PQRST

Rationale:

Correct answer: B

The acronym REEDA is often a scale used to assess the perineum when there is an episiotomy or laceration present. REEDA stands for:

R = Redness

E = Edema

E = Ecchymosis

D = Discharge

A = Approximation

A is incorrect because BUBBLE-LE is an acronym helpful for remembering the components of the general postpartum assessment; Breasts, Uterus, Bowel function, Bladder, Lochia, Episiotomy/perineum, Lower extremities, Emotions.

*It should be noted that in the past, the acronym was BUBBLE-HE, with the H representing Homan's sign, however, current best evidence has found that Homan's sign is unreliable, insensitive, and non-specific as an assessment for deep-vein-thrombosis.

C is incorrect because HELLP is associated with signs of severe preeclampsia: Hemolysis, Elevated Liver function, Low Platelet count.

D is incorrect because PQRST assists with pain assessment, asking: what Provokes the pain; what is the Quality of the pain; does the pain Radiate; what is the Severity of the pain; and what is the Timing of the pain?

24. Which of these findings, if identified during postpartum assessment at 4-6 hours past birth, would indicate that the patient is at risk for developing a complication?

    E. Temperature 100.2°F (37.9°C)
    F. Urinary output of 90 mL per 4-hr void
    G. Blood pressure 98/52 mm/Hg

H. Heart rate 60 beats per minute

Rationale:

Correct answer: B

Urinary output should be at least 30-60 mL per hour. Voiding 90 mL in 4 hours could be a sign of urinary retention related to compromised bladder tone that may occur after giving birth.

A is incorrect because temperature up to 100.4°F (38°C) is expected after delivery. The woman's body, regardless of vaginal or caesarean delivery, has experienced a traumatic event, and the typical immune response is expected, including a slightly elevated body temperature and slightly elevated white blood cells count. *Note: an increasing temperature or WBC count postpartum is indicative of infection.

C is incorrect because the BP is within normal limits for the postpartum period. BP between 90/50 and 140/90 is expected after birth.

D is incorrect because a somewhat slowed heart rate, between 50-70 beats per minute, is common after delivery, especially if the mother was athletic or in good physical shape, to begin with. Nonetheless, HR of 60 BPM is within normal limits.

25. Assessment strategies to identify whether a postpartum patient is developing a deep vein thrombosis (DVT) include which of the following? Select all that apply.

   A. Placing the patient's knee in an extended position and forcefully dorsiflexing the patient's foot
   B. Palpation of pedal pulses, noting color and temperature
   C. Examination of the lower extremities for the presence of hot, red, painful, and/or edematous areas
   D. Taking the patient's temperature
   E. Comparison of lower leg diameters

Rationale:

Correct answer: B, C, D, E

Assessment of the lower extremities for DVT includes palpation of pedal pulses, noting color and temperature, and examination for the presence of hot, red, painful areas, or edema. An elevated temperature may also be present with DVT. Difference in lower leg diameter may also indicate unilateral swelling, which can also be a characteristic finding of DVT.

A is incorrect because, in the past, assessment for DVT included eliciting Homans' sign: the presence of pain elicited with forceful passive dorsiflexion of the foot.

Current best evidence has found that Homan's sign is unreliable, insensitive, and non-specific as an assessment for deep-vein-thrombosis, and may be dangerous, related to a potential for clot mobilization throughout the body, which can contribute to pulmonary embolism or cerebral blood clot.

Made in United States
Orlando, FL
18 February 2022

14944465R00070